Body Balance

Proven Guide To Holistic Self-Care
and Supporting Your Health

Table of Content

Introduction

They say "health is wealth" and it is definitely true because without the presence of wellness every part of your life can go wrong. You can have all the money in the world but without good health, everything will be useless although you can cure some of the illnesses if you have a lot of money not all of them can be cured successfully such as cancer and other chronic diseases like diabetes and hypertension.

There are too many illnesses to mention that does not guarantee a complete cure even you have a lot of money that is why turning into a holistic way of living is very important.

How did I say so? Maybe you are wondering what is my capacity to guide you all throughout if I am not a medical practitioner, simply because I have experienced almost all the unimaginable things that you might encounter when you are struggling for health.

But I am very fortunate that I have surpassed those challenges on the dark years of my life.

To give you a brief background about myself I am a middle-aged guy which is very sickly since I was a child it is just recently wherein I discovered the benefits of a holistic lifestyle.

Since then I became healthy once again and all my previous illnesses have disappeared eventually. But my path towards wellness isn't an easy one as I have tried a lot of ways but eventually failed. However, my motivation towards wellness is really exceptional that is why I did not give up even though I am failing until then I found the ways on how to do the holistic lifestyle properly.

As a sign of gratitude, I will be sharing to you with the help of this book the knowledge that I learned throughout the years on achieving a healthy body. So let us not delay the learning and I would like to impart the learning immediately on the proceeding chapters of this book. I hope that you will learn a lot from this and apply the knowledge in your daily life.

Chapter 1 – Battling My Health Issues

Any of us suffer from different health issues and we all need different kinds of medication in order to heal or somehow relieve the pain we're feeling. Some of us go on the typical type of medication which is conventional medicine but others rely on alternative medicine which is more convenient because it only includes yourself and the things that will heal you.

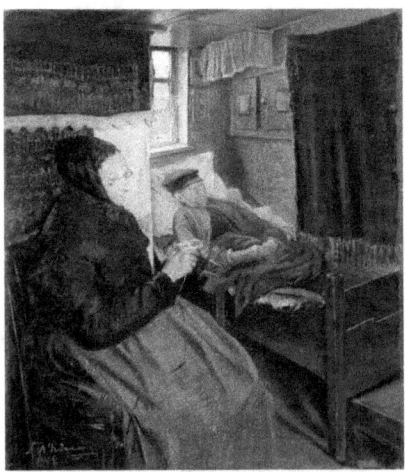

No matter what type of medication we use or we tend to believe in, one must still be aware of his/her health condition.

Start having a good lifestyle, exercise every morning, eat healthy foods or organic foods and try avoiding the processed ones, in this way you'll be having a much healthier lifestyle, not only it will make you strong and fit but will also make you feel very comfortable of your surroundings, having a less thought of an unhealthy lifestyle.

The main thing is, you need to believe or somehow convince yourself that you can do it, and the use of medicines are supplementary and the whole healing process is within you.

How did I say so? Because when I was still young I am very sickly particularly with my respiratory and skin problems that is why I am really depressed before as a child because my performance was stunted by my illnesses.

The turning point of my life is when I felt that I am very fed up with the situation and could not manage to stay a little bit longer on it.

So I looked for different ways to become healthy in order for me not to experience the same feeling that I felt when I was still sickly.

Thankfully, after several trial and errors, I found the different routines that will help us people in maintaining a healthy and sound body. This is what we will tackle all throughout in this book that is why brace yourselves of the knowledge that you will learn here.

Honestly, before the word "holistic" is an alien word to me as I do not have any idea on the meaning of it. When the worst period of came by wherein I became frequently ill this is the only time that I became aware that I must take good care of my health, in short, it was a good "wake up call."

The good thing with the holistic approach is that it does not have any side-effects that are why I really liked it among all the different types of the healing process.

Although, I experienced a lot of trial and error before I was lucky that I was able to formulate these routines myself to heal my illnesses and make my body stronger.

On the next chapter, we will tackle carefully on what is the difference between the medical way and the holistic way before we go to the latter part which is the routine itself.

Chapter 2 – Medical Intervention versus Holistic Way

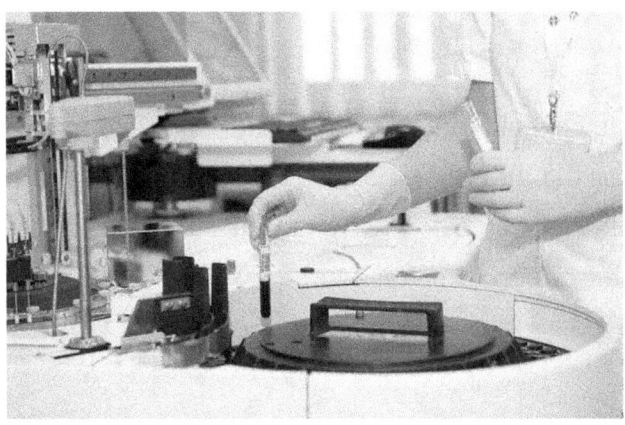

When it comes to medication we often think of the most basic thing to do when we are sick, consult a doctor right? Then right after get the prescribed medicines to treat our illness. But do you ever wonder what kind of treatments are used on us patients by the doctors? In this chapter, we'll be discussing the three most common medicine systems physicians used. First is the holistic medicine, holistic medicine is more of a philosophy than an actual treatment as it comes from the word "Holism" which means that parts of a whole are interconnected with each other and works as a whole.

The same thing in holistic medicine, it is a belief that a person's illness is caused by disharmony in the system of the whole body itself. It is also believed in holistic medicine that a person is capable of healing him/herself using the mind, body, and spirit. In holistic medicine, not only the illness is cured but it focuses more on the whole body itself, making it adaptable to any illness.

The idea of holistic medicine is more like taking care of yourself. As an example, nowadays the trend of D.I.Y. things can really save you a lot of time and most of all, convenient, it is one of the ideas that support holistic medicine, people tend to make their own treatments rather than to consult a doctor. It's true that the time you've invested waiting for a doctor in the hospital can be the time that you're already making your own remedies at home. All in all, holistic medicine is more about the way of living, a lifestyle rather than your usual medical treatment.

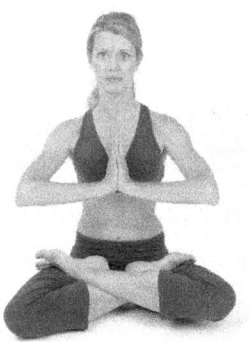

Next in line is the alternative medicine, so what is alternative medicine really? Well, in short terms these are the kind of treatments that use natural or traditional medicines. There are different types of alternative medicines and I am going to list down three in order for you to have furthermore understanding, these three are the Traditional Chinese Medicine, Homeopathy and Herbalism. Let us start with the Traditional Chinese Medicine, often compared with homeopathy (I'll explain later why), the word itself says 'Traditional' which means that this alternative medicine was discovered thousands of years ago.

It focuses more on the body healing itself and commonly the diagnosis is based on the doctor's personal observation of the patient then he/she will make the treatment to heal the person itself and not the illness.

Often criticized due to the principle this treatment follows and that is the diagnosis of the doctor based on the personal observation and not conducting a more precise examination. This lead people to question the treatment's effectiveness. There is also another factor that this treatment is being criticized with and it is about the ingredients used in making the medicine which is not scientifically proven effective.

The next type of alternative medicine is herbalism, it is obvious that this kind of treatment came from our ancestors. This only shows the early humans' creativeness in making medicines, they used different types of herbs, flowers, and plants in order to make a medicine that can cure a certain illness, although back then they do not have the advanced technology we have, they are certain that their medicines will work.

Hard to believe right? But back then it really works, maybe because it is the only thing they can find in their surroundings and that their bodies adapted on the medicines they make that is why it works, but now many people find this topic debatable as they think if this kind of treatment is still viable these days despite having the advanced technology. It is kind of ironic hearing people complain about the effectiveness of these alternative medicines the same time questions the safety in using advanced medical systems or treatments, like for example the CT scans, they're afraid of the radiation.

Last alternative medicine we're going to discuss is the homeopathy. It is a treatment that believes in the principle "likes cure likes" which means that if a substance is applied to a person in large amounts it will show symptoms of illness and by applying a small amount of the same substance will heal the illness. It also believes in the principle that the treatment is more effective if the substance is diluted, which means that the substance must be properly diluted first in order for it to take effect.

But one must be cautious in using this kind of
medication as it was discovered almost hundreds of
years ago and there is insufficient evidence that this
kind of treatment works and safe. Some scientists
argued that it only works because people are more
likely convincing themselves that it'll work, more
like the saying "To see is to believe." Having the
right mind setting together with solid evidence
(alternative medicine) to work on with, well I must
say people will really believe that it will heal them.
Now here it is, homeopathy is most likely compared
to traditional Chinese medicine as it both believes
in the principle: "the body is healing and not the
illness itself."

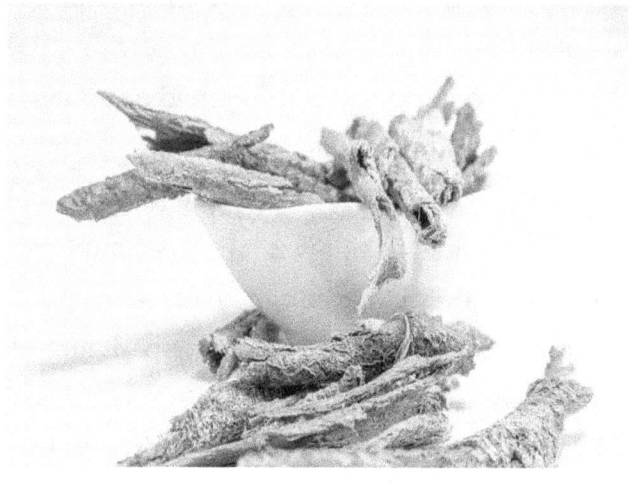

The final medical system we're going to discuss is the Complementary Medicine. Complementary medicine is the use of medical therapies in order to heal a patient, and any practitioner on this field must have proper training and certification as it provides complexity in performing, and one must be careful. There are types of complementary medicine, most of these are very common and in a way we enjoy them, I am again listing down three of them and we'll start with Chiropractic.

So basically what is Chiropractic? Often believed it started in the year 2000s until the present, it started way back on the 19th century. This therapy offers a technique called spinal manipulative therapy, it is a therapy that is performed on spinal articulations. Some doctor debates on the effectiveness of chiropractic but people tend to afford this treatment as they can avoid certain surgeries which they believed can be cured by chiropractic leads doctors in suggesting patients consult a chiropractor before starting surgery. The main reason why people tend to go on chiropractors is for back or neck pain, they depend mostly on spinal manipulative therapy.

It doesn't show much evidence that it actually cures an illness as it only brings back joints to its original place especially when they're dislocated, others claim that they suffer from side effects after chiropractic, which made other insurance companies not pay for chiropractic service due to the effectiveness of chiropractic.

Second complementary medicine is the most enjoyable, for me personally, the massage therapy. It manipulates soft tissues in the body giving a pleasurable feeling when performed, this treatment usually releases stress and pain from the body. Massage Therapy is obviously the most common complementary medicine, there are still things scientists debate about this treatment and one of them is the relief it gives. Maybe it'll give you a pleasurable and enjoyable experience it is not guaranteed that it will give you long term of pain relief. From time to time, massage became a universal treatment not only to relieve pain temporarily but it also made its way to the scientists becoming less doubtful about the long term effects of massage therapy. Now it can also cure people with depression, anxiety, cancer, and other serious illness.

The last complementary medicine that we'll discuss is the Acupuncture, titled one of the most famous treatments in Traditional Chinese Medicine, acupuncture made its way to the western countries. The procedure in performing acupuncture is a bit odd, it uses different sizes of needles and then inserted into the body, specifically on what they called 'meridians' which they believe the pathways of the energy flowing to inside the body. It is believed that piercing through these vital points can heal a person with chronic back pain, arthritis and many more kinds of illness. Like its other affiliates, many still debates about the acupuncture's effectiveness often believed as a pseudoscience due to lack of scientific evidence, people still tend to believe on its efficacy which made it famous up to this day.

A Broader Explanation of the Inclusion of Holistic Medicine into Conventional Medicine

Despite the doubts, conventional medicines have on alternative medicines due to its efficacy and safety, it still made its way on conventional medicine.

Western medical schools already started teaching alternative medicine on their students as a part of conventional medicine. There is no doubt that the alternative medicine will stand out, this is because of the holistic ideology on it, people tend to do things on their own when it comes to their health rather than to trust scientific doctors. Not only it will 'heal' the person but it will also balance the person's state of mind, emotionally and spiritually which conventional medicine does not offer. Having alternative medicine in conventional medical training allows doctors to understand and communicate with his/her patients thoroughly. This gives an advantage to conventional medical doctors. The last thing to understand is that having the knowledge in alternative medicine included in conventional medicine will make patients understand and believe its efficacy because it is now scientifically related, but in reality still not that proven.

Being allowed to be practiced, there are still limitations in distributing the knowledge in alternative medicine because the first thing is still followed and it's the patient's safety.

Chapter 3 – My Holistic Self-Care Tips

The word itself, holistic pertains to the union of the parts of a whole. That only means for you to have a well and healthy perfect working body, you must work out your way through in enhancing different parts of your body for them to function as one. These include the three elements in holistic care, your physical, emotional and spiritual health.

Obtaining such a healthy body doesn't mean that it is only within you, it also talks about the environment you are living in, is it clean? Non-toxic? And many more factors in your surroundings that may affect your health. But somehow it is unbelievable to free ourselves from toxins, why? Simple, because every day we're exposed in pollution, different chemicals flying around that came from smoke and not only in the surroundings, also in foods, chemicals are often found in foods especially the processed ones.

But hey! You don't need to worry, despite this factors you might think that it is almost impossible to have a perfectly healthy lifestyle but no, you can still have the lifestyle you've been dreaming for (obviously the healthy one).

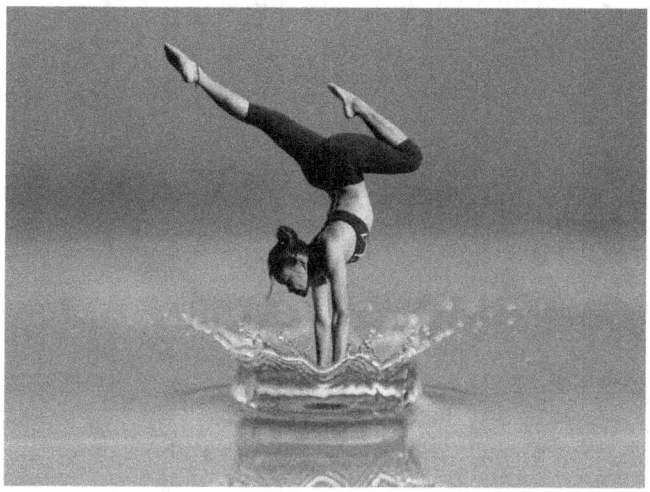

There are different ways you can achieve a healthy and fit body, starting with your physical health, you may hear of this word a lot, 'diet'. Yes, you heard it right! Diet is the most common thing when it comes to physical health, diet does not only about the exercises you do every day, how much weight you've been losing, and etc.

But it also tells about the food you eat, in order to possess a fit body and healthy the same time, you must reduce the intake of processed foods as much as possible and turning on eating organic foods. I didn't mean to say you must be a vegan in order to achieve the lifestyle you want, but you need to balance things out in order for your desired outcome to become true.

Have you ever heard of the word 'probiotics'? For common knowledge, these are bacteria, yep you heard it right again, bacteria, but it is not your typical bacteria that cause disease, it is more of a "good" bacteria". Just for a fact, we all have bacteria inside our body it is a balance of "good" and "bad" bacteria. When your body loses these "good" bacteria, probiotics are an essential thing to have in order to return those good bacteria in your body, keeping the balance within you. For further knowledge, I'll be listing down the health benefits of probiotics.

First thing is, probiotics produce B vitamins which are essential in the digestive cycle, second thing is they make your immune system more adaptable and strong, they also produce a certain substance called "lactase" that helps in digesting dairy products, they protect your body for radiation and gets rid of the toxins that may harm your body. Probiotics are also essential in reducing high cholesterol levels in your body and serves as an anti-bacterial agent that kills bad bacteria which cause diseases.

Now done with the knowledge about the foods and healthy substances that can help you, next thing we're going to discuss about the holistic routine is exercise. You need to have a daily routine to follow in order to fulfill your desire in having a healthy lifestyle, this includes the basic warm-ups, weightlifting, jogging, taking your dog for a walk, and the right cooldowns after. Having an hour and a half every day for exercise can help you a lot, so yeah, choose the exercises that are right for you and not against your free will and you'll not regret the outcome it'll give you.

Adding up in a healthy lifestyle, sleep plays an important role. It is said that you must have at least 8 hours of sleep every day as it will reserve your body for work the next day, and not just that, it will balance your sleep cycle and make you healthier.

Now for the second part of the holistic self-care, mental health is now up on the list. Your mental health also plays an important role in your holistic lifestyle because what's the sense of having a perfect body without the right mindset? I'll be giving tips on how to maintain your mental health.

1. Having support from family and friends will give you a positive outlook in life that can help you keep your mental state healthy.
2. Did you know that practice in proper breathing is also a factor that affects your mental health? Yes, it does, so the best thing to do is start practicing the control in your breathing to keep your mental health properly.
3. Stressed? Write it down, some may find this tip boring but I assure you it works. Writing down your everyday experiences or at least writing down the things that stress you can help you lessen your stress.

4. Day off? Break time? Go on, relax. Relaxation is the most essential thing to do to cool your head from a stressful day and it's obvious, it'll surely make your mental health stable.

Last but not least in the holistic self-care is spiritual health. It is more about connecting yourself with your spirit. Reflecting through your soul is an effective way of enhancing your spiritual health. There are a lot of ways you can do this. First is to isolate yourself from the world and meditate, in this way you're calm and you can achieve your peace of mind giving you a right amount of time in reflecting, second thing is spending time with your family and friends, enjoying each moment with close ties can be a good source in the enhancement of one's spiritual health. Also if you're the person who has his/her time, you can go volunteer on different charities, in this way, you're positive emotions and mental healthiness will increase together with your spiritual health.

So far we're glad to give you these tips in holistic self-care. Knowing this information can help you a lot and now it is up to you to act on it. Good luck in achieving the healthy lifestyle you've always wanted!

The path to Long Lasting Happiness and Well-Being with the use of Holistic Self-Care

For a person to fulfill his/her desires in achieving long-lasting happiness and well-being, he/she must have self-realization, reflections on everyday experiences. And one must look in maintain the balance in life and not having less or too much. There are aspects in life we can look out for and maintain properly and these are the physical, intellectual, emotional, social, and spiritual aspect. We'll be listing down ways to keep these aspects in good condition:

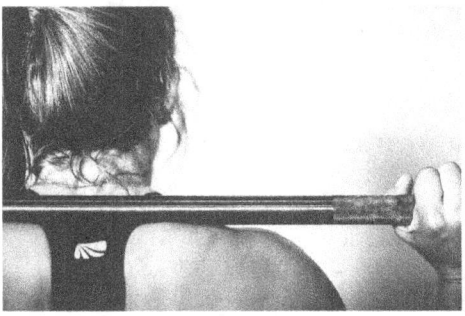

- Physical
  - ➢ Having enough rest every day is a must as it gives time for the body to heal and refresh from stress and hard work.

- Eating healthy foods and avoiding processed ones.
- Having a daily routine, like exercising.
- Waking up 7:00 am in the morning to get sufficient Vitamin D from the sun.
- Avoiding any vices, especially the most common one: Alcohol

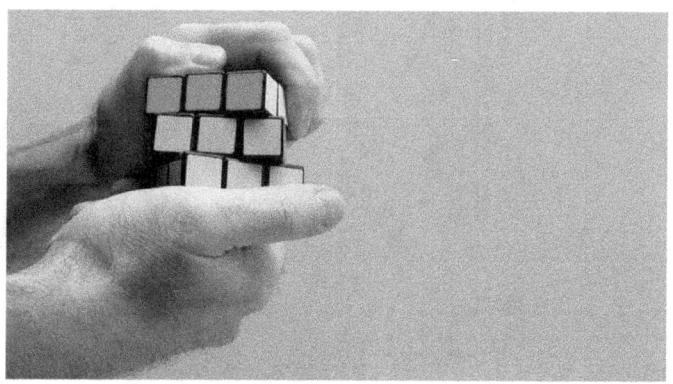

- Intellectual
  - Having reflexive thinking.
  - Having yourself teachable with new things.
  - Getting the right education.
  - Reading books, articles, newspapers and other literary works.

- Traveling in different places to expand your knowledge about the place's culture.
- Writing down your experiences in a journal.
- Being organized in planning things you want to do in a week.

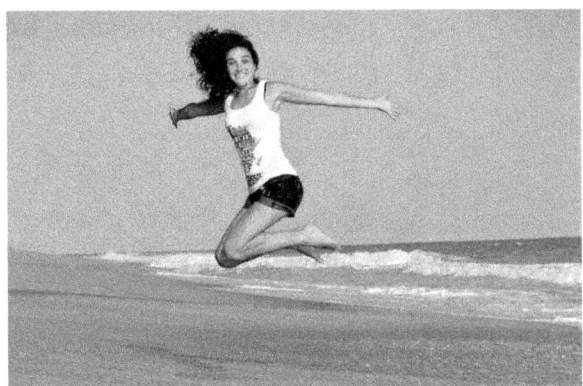

- Emotional
  - Smile!
  - Don't over think!
  - Be proactive and less reactive on things.
  - Have a positive outlook in life even on your darkest days, because after all, it'll be alright.
  - Fulfilling your promises to people.
  - Being content on things you have, keeping it simple.

- Controlling and understanding your own emotions.
- Dealing with other's mood change.
- Staying away from toxic relationships.
- Believe in yourself!
- Don't judge other people because you don't like it you being judged, but hey who cares if others judge you right? You know yourself better than them.

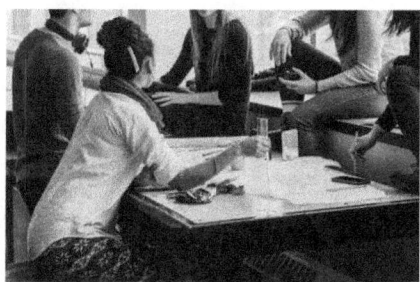

- Social
  - Spend time outside your home and start socializing with people personally.
  - Spend time for your family and friends.
  - Practicing good manners.
  - Often say thank you and please.
  - Be concern in your surroundings.

- Work voluntarily.
- Avoiding disagreements in a certain topic with other people and finding similarities instead.
- Support other people when you can and at the same time accept the support that is being offered to you.
- Sharing your problem with a close friend or vice versa, listen to their problems.
- Be a good listener, understanding what you have listened is really important too.

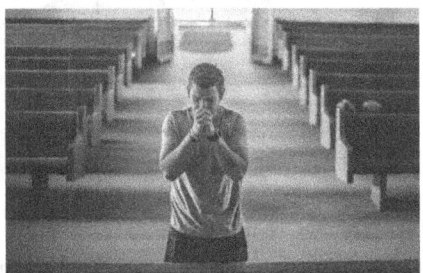

- Spiritual
  - Giving yourself time to silently reflect.
  - Having time to meditate.
  - Practicing being calm in any situation.

- ➢ Indulge yourself in music or arts.
- ➢ Following your heart, often listen to yourself and trust yourself.
- ➢ Do good things without recognition.
- ➢ Being thankful for all the good things you have in life.
- ➢ Reading positive quotes.
- ➢ Stop running and start facing all your fears.
- ➢ Love!
- ➢ Having your own mission in life which you are committed to fulfill.

Following these guides can lead you to long-lasting happiness and enhance your well-being.

Chapter 4 – My Holistic Routines and Diets

There are some people lucky enough to live in rural places provided with natural and organic food for a healthier lifestyle. The urban community is often deprived by this

because factories are the most common industrial structure you can see there (food factories to be exact). People living in rural areas may not enjoy the burgers in the urban areas but they do enjoy a much healthier lifestyle and that's a huge difference.

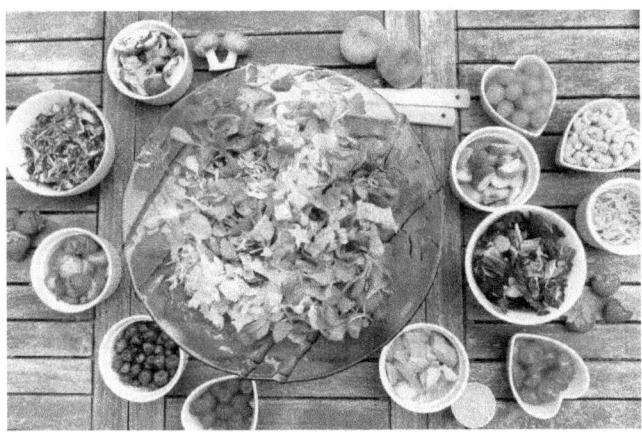

There are a lot of factors affecting the urban residen ts which gave them a hard time providing themselv es with healthy foods, some of these factors are the quality and price of the healthy food, the distance of their houses on the grocery store, and the quantity of the healthy foods being supplied in their local ma rkets.

There are some communities that made their way t o fight back chronic diseases by creating different st rategies. Their approach in increasing the physical a ctivity and healthy food consumption is superb, tak e for an example, Philadelphia, it has been reported that there is a 4.7% decrease in obesity among child ren by having an increase in healthy food consumpt ion. That's why Philadelphia doubled their program , making groceries near neighborhoods so that they can be provided by the right amount of healthy food s and nutrition education.

A sound eating routine is a place everything begins. Today, there is so much data accessible about sound weight control plans it is difficult to try and make sense of – What precisely is a solid eating regimen? Everybody may have their very own meaning of what that is on the grounds that every last one of us is so unique.

Where a specific eating regimen can do some amazing things for one individual it can likewise make someone else feel horrible.

This is my meaning of a solid eating regimen:

- Loads of natural vegetables – you'll have to try for yourself whether crude or cooked works best.

- Solid fats – olive oil, coconut oil, crude natural spread (in the event that you endure dairy) and stay away from vegetable oils

- Fed meats and eggs – not manufacturing plant cultivated or handled and originated from the moral and economical practice

- Wild gotten fish

- Beans and vegetables – drenched (whenever endured)

- Natural crude nuts and seeds

- Custom made stocks, juices and soups – vegetable, chicken, meat, fish, and so on. Figure out how to make bone soup or Veggie stock

- Natural organic products (in season)

- Low grain, no grain, doused or grew grain, or sourdough – experimentation will reveal to you what works for you.

- Organic foods and drinks – fermented tea, water kefir, sauerkraut, pickles, and so forth.

- Maintain a strategic distance from gluten.

- Maintain a strategic distance from refined sugar – stick to nectar, maple syrup, dates, and stevia

- Maintain a strategic distance from bundled and prepared nourishments

- Maintain a strategic distance from regular dairy items

Remember these focuses and you will surely have better overall health that will lead to better performance. Although they might be a lot for some to memorize my advice is to take down some notes on a sticky notepad and put it on your wall or wherever you can easily see it.

This will help you to be reminded of your responsibilities as a person to your whole body. This is the best technique that you can do in order to stay on track because from time to time as people tend to get bored easily on the routines that they are doing.

Conclusion

What a great ride! I hope that you learned a lot from the techniques and routines that we tackled in this book. As long as you put the knowledge that you learned to your heart and apply it in your life meticulously you will surely reap the benefits of this holistic lifestyle. I know this is not an overnight process but the benefits of it can surpass the amount that you will pay for if you got sick and the experiences that you will miss.

I am truly looking forward to your massive improvements with regards to health as we go on with our daily lives, your health is your number one weapon. Now you already know the techniques you can be pretty confident that you will become better on all the aspects of your life as well.

Although you already know the techniques it will not work if you do not have the discipline and perseverance to continue implementing it on a day to day basis. Just what other kinds of things that you are doing it is very important to commit yourself into it in order for you to achieve success this is the primary secret as you will not reap the benefits if you are a quitter.So I wish you good luck and health, wish you all the best as well on your future endeavors